Detox Cleanse Made Easy – A Complete Home Guide on How to Detoxify

Be Young, Sexy and Healthy

By: Joan Evans

9781634289740

PUBLISHERS NOTES

Disclaimer – Speedy Publishing LLC

This publication is intended to provide helpful and informative material. It is not intended to diagnose, treat, cure, or prevent any health problem or condition, nor is intended to replace the advice of a physician. No action should be taken solely on the contents of this book. Always consult your physician or qualified health-care professional on any matters regarding your health and before adopting any suggestions in this book or drawing inferences from it.

The author and publisher specifically disclaim all responsibility for any liability, loss or risk, personal or otherwise, which is incurred as a consequence, directly or indirectly, from the use or application of any contents of this book.

Any and all product names referenced within this book are the trademarks of their respective owners. None of these owners have sponsored, authorized, endorsed, or approved this book.

Always read all information provided by the manufacturers' product labels before using their products. The author and publisher are not responsible for claims made by manufacturers.

This book was originally printed before 2014. This is an adapted reprint by Speedy Publishing LLC with newly updated content designed to help readers with much more accurate and timely information and data.

Speedy Publishing LLC

40 E Main Street, Newark, Delaware, 19711

Contact Us: 1-888-248-4521

Website: http://www.speedypublishing.co

REPRINTED Paperback Edition: ISBN: 9781634289740

Manufactured in the United States of America

DEDICATION

I dedicate this book to all those who are dreaming of becoming healthy, fit, and sexy. This book will tell you how and start living a toxin free life!

TABLE OF CONTENTS

Publishers Notes..2

Dedication 3

Table of Contents..4

Chapter 1- Let's Understand Body Detoxification 5

Chapter 2- Body Detoxification is Essential and Needed 10

Chapter 3- Questions on the Regularities in Detoxifying 15

Chapter 4- Body Detoxification – A Great Way to Shed Off Some Fats 20

Chapter 5- How Does Detoxification Help in Losing Weight?.....28

Chapter 6- Recipes for Home-made Detox Drinks 38

Chapter 7- Addiction and the Role of Detoxification.....................52

Chapter 8- Detoxification and Choosing the Right Nutrition to Beat Addiction 55

Chapter 9- Detoxifying Addiction Away 58

About The Author..63

CHAPTER 1- LET'S UNDERSTAND BODY DETOXIFICATION

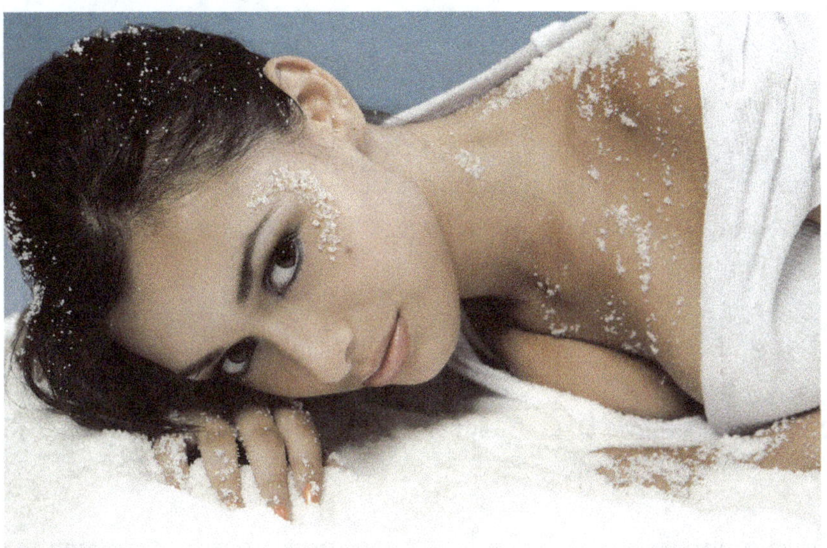

Detoxification is a process by which you'll remove the toxic elements from your body in order to restore your health. Your body undergoes a lot of wear and tear throughout your day to day life. Toxins and free radicals are affecting your organs, your skin and your overall well being on the inside and on the outside.

During the course of your normal daily life, you could be exposed to harsh chemicals through your work environment. You could be ingesting harmful ingredients in your food. All of these elements working together can cause a very toxic environment in your body.

Once you get to understand about body detoxification and how it works, however, you will have a different opinion.

Body detoxification concentrates on cleaning out your digestive system, usually by drinking a solution that is made to clear out your intestines and give the organs in your digestive system a boost. Although it may sound like a surgical procedure, body detoxification only involves drinking and then going to the bathroom. That is all there is to the procedure. It works to make sure that your digestive system is healthy.

Things like cigarettes, acidic foods, caffeine, junk food and soda are all harmful to your health. If you are consuming these things on a consistent basis, you are harming your body on several levels. All of these elements build up in your system over time and can cause a whole host of problems including weight gain, memory problems and immune system issues.

Detoxification is a natural process that the body accomplishes all on it's own under normal circumstances. However, when you have a poor diet and a stressful lifestyle your body isn't able to cleanse your system properly.

If your body is not able to do its job properly, you can take steps to help your body heal itself.

Detoxification can:

- Improve your immune system function
- Eliminate free radicals from your system
- Improve your ability to fight off cancer cells
- Cleanse out congestion and mucous from your body
- Purify your blood
- Help you break your addiction to sugar, salt, alcohol and junk foods

Detoxification is slowly being acknowledged by modern medicine, but there are still skeptics out there. In this report, we'll go over the most popular detoxification products in addition to some more natural methods of detoxification that will help you lose weight and get the rest of the benefits from detoxification.

When your digestive system is in good working order, your whole body sings. If your digestive system is not healthy, then your whole body suffers. In order to have a healthy body, you must have a healthy digestive system.

But your digestive system is the catch all for all of the toxins that you take into your body. Even if you are a healthy person who does not smoke, does not drink and eats only organic foods, you are still taking in toxins. They are in the air that you breathe the water that you drink and....well, just about everywhere. These toxins linger in the body and find their way to the digestive system - a vital system that you need to maintain good health.

The digestive system is comprised of organs such as the liver, pancreas, kidneys and intestines. Foods usually enter the digestive system through the stomach and are then passed for processing through the digestive tract. Some foods and drinks that you take in make the kidneys and pancreas work overtime in processing them. All of the organs in the digestive system have a job to do in order to keep your body running healthy. Once food and drink is processed in the system, it is then eliminated by way of waste. Liquids are eliminated by urine and solid waste is eliminated through the intestines as feces.

In some cases, foods can end up getting stuck in the intestines. There are cases where people have had elements in their intestines for 10 years! In addition, the organs also take a beating when it comes to getting rid of toxins as well as some foods that can be difficult for these organs to process. Simple carbohydrates, for example, are very hard on the kidneys and pancreas as well as the liver as they tend to pass through quickly and make these organs work overtime.

Toxins in the air that you breathe enter the system through the circulatory system that brings blood to and from the organs. When you smoke, for example, the smoke is absorbed into your bloodstream and carried throughout your body. This negatively affects the digestive system. Even second hand smoke will take its toll.

Your skin is your biggest organ and when you take a bath or shower using chemicals as are featured in shampoo and soap, you are absorbing toxins into your skin. When you breathe in air, you take the toxins into your lungs. It is impossible to live your life toxin free, although a good many people try.

You are going to eventually go out and pick up germs that are in the air. It is inevitable that you will come into contact with toxins unless you decide to live your life in a plastic bubble body detoxification clears the body of all of the toxins and foods that sit in the digestive system. Not only is it a good way to get the poisons out of your body, but it also works well when it comes to losing weight. Most people find that they can take off quite a few pounds simply by using body detoxification.

Drinking body detoxification fluid is similar to taking a barium enema, except you do not have to drink as much and it tastes much better. A barium enema completely clears out your intestines and is usually given to those who are having tests done on their colon or other digestive organs. This eliminates all of the waste from the body and makes you feel lighter. Not only can it get rid of toxins, but it can get rid of any waste that is lingering in your intestines.

Drinking the body detoxification formula is one of the first steps towards being healthier. You should also take proper precautions when it comes to your health and eat right, exercise and avoid bad habits. Body detoxification should be seen as a way to enhance your health, help you lose weight and keep your digestive system healthy. Good body detoxification will also fill your body with the nutrients that you may be lacking so that you stay healthy as well.

This book will teach you all about body detoxification at home and what you need to know about this way of staying fit and healthy. You will learn about the different aspects of body detoxification, who should body cleanse and even how to make your own body detoxification treatments right at home. If you are looking for a way to lose weight, stay healthy and keep your digestive system in good working order, you can find it by embarking on body detoxification.

CHAPTER 2- BODY DETOXIFICATION IS ESSENTIAL AND NEEDED

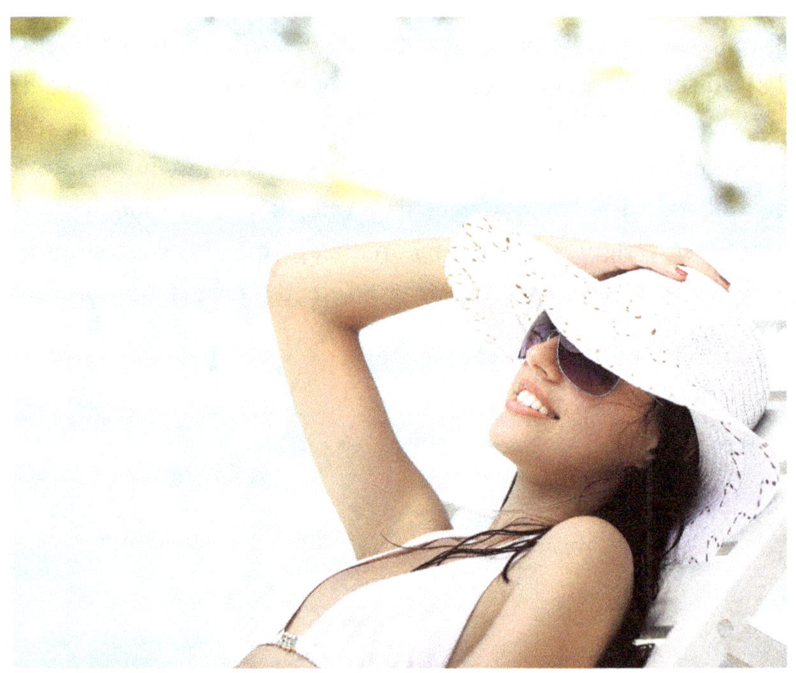

One of the primary reasons that people use home body detoxification is to detoxify their bodies. There are several products on the market that are made for body detoxification. These include products that range from those that can help you pass a drug test to those that can renew your body with organic herbs that rid your body of toxins that you may unwittingly take in.

Detoxification by body detoxification is usually done with a solution that you drink, although there are teas as well as tablets that you can take as well. Kits for home body detoxification often consist of tablets and teas as well as solutions that can be mixed in with water. It is often cheaper to buy these kits than to buy products that are already mixed together.

You should plan to use a body detoxifier to detoxify your body once a week if you have a lifestyle like most normal people that entails taking in toxins. You can mix up the remedy right at home and drink it. Most of the body detoxification kits that are sold online have pleasant taste to them and they will go to work right away to move through your system and ridding your body from toxins.

In addition to drinking the solution or taking the tablets, you will have to drink plenty of water. There are often instructions on how much water you should drink after you take the solution. Water will help the body detoxification product flush through your system and detoxify your body detoxification not only rids your body of impurities that are found in the air, foods and drinks but it also can rid your body of ailments. If you are trying to get over a cold, have stress or physical ailments, you will be surprised at how the body detoxification works to detoxify your system and make you feel better.

Choosing a home kit is the best option when you are seeking to body cleanse for health. This is not only the less expensive alternate, but it also allows you to use the kit whenever you feel the need to purify your body. The ingredients in the body detoxification kit should be all herbal ingredients that will work their way through your system and help you detoxify.

Drug Detox

If you are worried about passing a drug test, you can choose a body detoxification system that will cleanse any impurities from your body. This will work only if you are taking a urine drug test. There are several body detoxification agents that are on the market that will not only provide your body with nutrients, but will also color the urine so that it is not clear. The way that drug detox drinks work is that you drink them down and then follow them with several glasses of water. You have to do this a few hours before taking the drug test, although there are some that will work in less than an hour. After you drink several glasses of water in rapid succession, you will be able to take the test. Instead of your urine turning clear, as it would if you drink a lot of water at one time, it will have a yellowish tinge to it. The herbal remedies that are used in the drug detox body detoxification are not detectible by most drug tests.

No matter why you decide to detoxify yourself, you should be certain to use a body detoxification system that is all natural and does not contain any chemicals. Whether you use a tea, a tablet or a solution that is pre-made, you will feel good after you have cleansed your body in this way.

Tips on Body Detoxification in a Natural Way

Although there are many products on the market for home body detoxification, you can also work towards cleansing your body at home without any products. One of the best ways to start body detoxification is to drink purified water. You should consume 6-8 glasses of water per day in order to maintain good health. Many people do not drink enough water and end up paying for it with weight gain and storing toxins in their body. Water is the natural way to flush toxins out of your body.

You can tell if you are drinking enough water by the color of your urine. If you are getting enough water, the urine should be nearly clear. If your urine is dark, it means that you are not drinking enough water. While it is more concentrated in the morning when you first go to the bathroom, it should get clearer throughout the day. Many people do not like drinking a lot of water throughout the day because they do not have time to use the bathroom frequently, however, it is one of the ways you can purify your body naturally. By keeping yourself hydrated, you will start to notice that you are better able to maintain your weight or even lose weight.

Another factor in natural body detoxification has to do with the foods that you eat. When you are trying to body cleanse, you should eat foods that are high in vitamins and minerals and low in fat. Eating at least seven fruits and vegetables a day will help you detoxify your system. Some of the foods that you will want to add to your diet include fish, blueberries, cranberries and leafy greens. These all work towards making you healthier by providing your body with nutrients that you need to maintain good health. You have most likely heard the old adage that you are what you eat. This is not just a saying, but a true fact. Start by cutting out fats, fast foods, sodium, processed foods and sweets from your diet that add toxins.

There is a large variety of organic products that you can choose as well. Organic foods are developed without toxins such as artificial hormones and chemicals. Eating organic foods is one way to keep your body clear of impurities.

Exercise is also essential for body detoxification. You should perform cardiovascular exercises that will work up a sweat as well as relaxing exercises, such as yoga, to eliminate stress. Many people today complain of stress over work, home or money. Stress can play havoc on your body and natural body detoxification should try to eliminate stress as much as possible. Exercise is a natural way to not only get in shape and burn calories, but also to sweat out toxins.

Supplements can also help you cleanse your body. You should take a good multivitamin in order to naturally cleanse your body. This will help you get the vitamins and minerals that you may be missing in your daily diet.

It stands to reason that you should practice good health habits and avoid behavior that leads to toxins entering your body. Do not smoke, take drugs or drink alcohol. These are habits that are detrimental to your health and should be avoided.

Once you get into the habit of naturally cleansing your body, you will find that it not only gets easier, but that you start to feel healthier and look better. Your entire body will respond to natural body detoxification. It is not difficult to use body detoxification at home once you understand how. When you start to see and feel the results, it even gets easier.

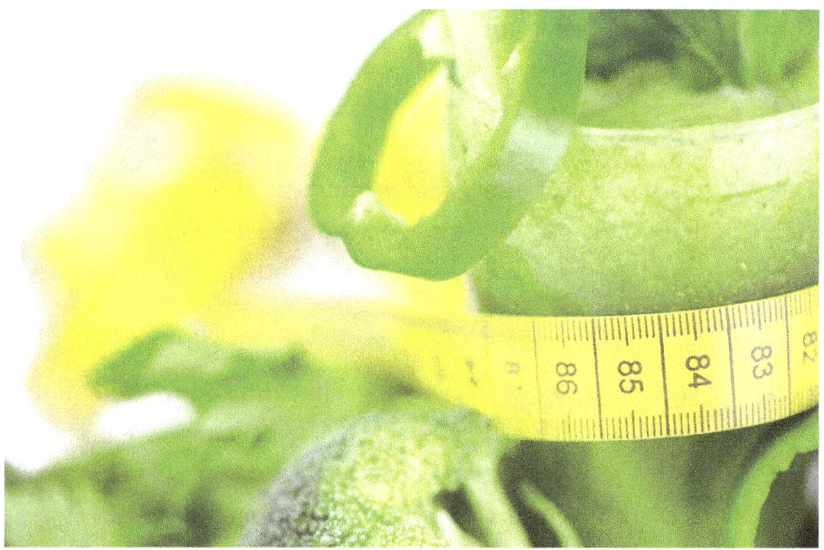

CHAPTER 3- QUESTIONS ON THE REGULARITIES IN DETOXIFYING

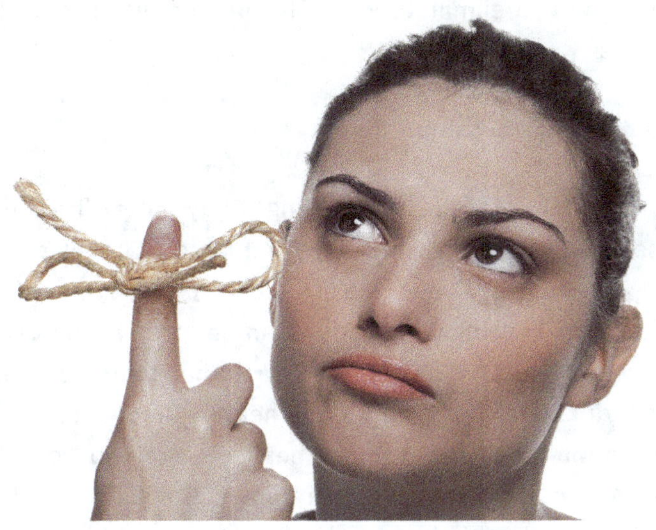

As stated earlier, just about anyone can make use of body detoxification. How often you use body detoxification materials depends on your lifestyle and the intent that you have for the body detoxification. If you want to lose weight, have a lifestyle that involves bad habits, such as smoking, you may want to use body detoxification more often. If you are just trying to maintain good digestive health, you can use body detoxification less often. But regardless of how often you decide to embark on this way to stay healthy, everyone needs body detoxification once in a while.

For Weight Loss

If you are trying to lose weight, you may want to try body detoxification. This will get rid of the waste in your body and you will feel much lighter. Many people who are looking for a way to lose weight opt for body detoxification. Body detoxification is one of the healthiest ways to lose weight.

Because you tend to store waste in your intestines, you may end up feeling bloated and retaining weight. Body detoxification eliminates the waste from your body and makes you feel lighter instantly. That being said, body detoxification is not a laxative. It is a natural way to eliminate waste from your system that leads to weight loss.

To Rid Yourself of Toxins

A lot of the celebrities are using body detoxification to rid themselves of toxins in which they imbibe on a regular basis. You can rid your body of toxins by using a body cleanse system. This will work towards keeping your body clean and free from poisons that are in what you consume as well as what you breathe. If you smoke, drink or do not always eat a healthy diet, you can use body detoxification as a way to stay healthier and rid your body of toxins. While body detoxification should not be a substitute for practicing good health, it can help alleviate the problems that come with taking in toxins.

Just about everyone comes into contact with toxins. Ridding the body of toxins by using body detoxification is not only good for the digestive system, but also good for overall health.

Keeping the Digestive System Healthy

Remember, your digestive system and its health is vital to the overall health of your body. Colon cancer, which is cancer of the small intestine, is the number 3 cancer killer in the United States. Colon cancer is the result of polyps in the colon. These polyps often result due to waste remaining in the colon. Body detoxification gets rid of the waste in the body and keeps the colon clean. On top of that, many body detoxification formulas have herbs, vitamins and minerals in them that can help the body detoxify the digestive system and can feed the organs with nutrients that are needed to keep it cleansed. A great many people use body detoxification as a way to maintain a healthy digestive system.

With natural body detoxification supplies, the body is fed a series of nutrients that not only end up helping the digestive system, but the rest of the body. The digestive organs send nutrients back through the body and to the heart, brain and other vital organs. Body detoxification cleans the entire body through the digestive organs.

Passing Drug Testing

Those who get drug tested for jobs often use body detoxification at home to remove the remnants of illegal substances from the body, such as marijuana. While body detoxification does not help with a drug blood test, it can help someone pass a urine test for illegal substances or even tobacco. Someone who imbibes on the weekend can end up passing a drug test on Monday by using body detoxification.

While it is not recommended that you use body detoxification as a way to use drugs and pass drug tests, it can help you if you happen to make a bad decision and then have to take a drug test. A lapse in sense does not have to cost you your job if you use body detoxification solutions that are made for passing drug tests.

There are many different body detoxification products on the market. Most of them are made to maintain good health. Others concentrate on cleansing toxins from the body or as a way to lose weight. Anyone who wants to maintain good health as well as lose weight can benefit from body detoxification solutions and tablets that are sold on the market.

When you are body detoxification at home, you can even create your own solutions using natural ingredients to cleanse your body. Later in this book, we will discuss home remedies, how to use them and even give you some recipes on how to make your own at home body detoxification formula.

While everyone can benefit from using body detoxification at home, this should never be considered as a substitute for common sense when it comes to health. While body detoxification can help you lose weight, rid your body of toxins, keep your colon clean and even help you pass a drug test, the best way to stay healthy is to avoid toxins, drugs, and eating the wrong foods. Natural at home body detoxification will also be discussed in a later chapter.

Colon Cleansing

A great many people who use body detoxification are interested in colon cleansing. These home body detoxification remedies can be used for eliminating constipation as well as making the colon healthy. Colon cleansing will eliminate any waste that you have in your body and clean it out.

Like the other body detoxification remedies, you can get colon cleansing in drink, tea or tablet form. There are also many kits that are used on the market for colon cleansing. Again, it is important to chase the solution or tablet with water so that it can make its way through your system.

There are various colon cleansing recipes and products that you can find on the internet. The ideal time to use colon cleansing is when you have time to relax and take the solution as well as have access to the bathroom. After colon cleansing works on you, you will feel lighter and more energetic. A great many people use colon cleansing as a way to lose weight as well. Most of the colons cleansing solutions are interchangeable with the weight loss solutions for body detoxification. They not only flush out the colon, but they also provide the body with treatment to keep the colon healthy.

There are many disease of the colon that can range from being inconvenient to being life threatening. One way to keep your colon healthy as well as maintain your weight is to use a colon cleanses body detoxification solution.

You can use a colon cleanse that you purchase at a health food store or online, or make your own. As is the case with all body detoxification, the key ingredient is water. In addition to water, you will want to add some natural products to help cleanse the colon and flush out the system. For colon cleansing, you should concentrate on using antioxidants that will not only help with colon cleansing, but will also help with health. One remedy that works well is pure grape juice mixed with water. This should not include the store bought grape juice, however, as it is filled with sugar. Resveratrol is also a supplement that can help with colon health as well as health of the entire digestive system. This is derived from the skin of red grapes. You can mix Resveratrol powder with water to make a colon cleanse that is healthy for colon health.

No matter what type of diet you consume, colon cleansing is a good way to keep the digestive system in good health. Whether you make your own solution or purchase a solution, you should use a colon cleanse once a week for good digestive health.

CHAPTER 4- BODY DETOXIFICATION – A GREAT WAY TO SHED OFF SOME FATS

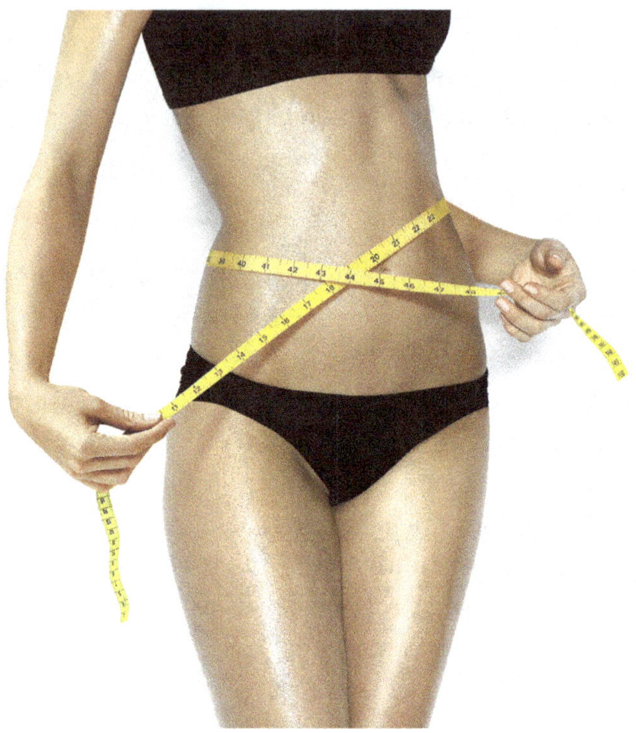

Losing weight can be difficult, especially if you want to take the pounds off fast. One way that you can use at home body detoxification is to help you lose those extra pounds. You can provide your body with nutrients and vitamins it needs to function while at the same time lose weight.

There are several solutions on the market as well as pills that can help you lose weight by body detoxification. The main ingredient that you need is water. You can use herbal supplements along with vitamins to help you lose weight with body detoxification. You can also use pre-made solutions that you purchase online or in health food stores as a body detoxification weight loss remedy.

Drinking plenty of water is one of the safest ways to lose weight. Water not only hydrates your system, but also fills you up and helps you expel excess water. You should drink 8 glasses of water a day whether or not you are trying to lose weight. Water is even more essential when you are trying to lose weight.

Water alone, however, is not sufficient when it comes to losing weight. You need to supply your body with nutrients, especially if you are skipping meals. On top of that, you need to cleanse the digestive tract so that waste is eliminated. You should look for body detoxification supplements that will provide your body with the essential vitamins it needs while helping you lose weight.

Body detoxification is the safe way to lose weight fast. Instead of taking weight loss pills that often contain illegal pharmaceutical ingredients, you can take off the weight with a body detoxification system. You can create your own body detoxification by mixing water with ingredients such as lemon and pepper that will cleanse out your system. There are also commercial brands of weight loss body detoxification products that you can purchase.

Using the body detoxification systems to lose weight is safer than diet drinks that act as laxatives and contain chemicals. When you are looking for a body detoxification solution to help you lose weight, look for one that has all natural ingredients instead of one that is filled with chemicals as this will not only help you lose weight, but will also be healthier for your body.

Green tea is one of the key components when it comes to weight loss through body detoxification. Green tea acts like a diuretic and can help you lose weight quicker. You should drink green tea without sugar in order to get the effects. Drink plenty of green tea a day and you will find that you are taking off the pounds. Green tea can also be taken in tablet form if you dislike the taste.

Cranberry also works as a diuretic and can help you lose weight through body detoxification. Cranberry should be used in tablet form as the juice drinks that you purchase in the grocery store are loaded with sugar. Cranberry will also help clean out your urinary tract.

There are many kits on the market that you can use to create your own home body detoxification solutions that enable you to lose weight. These include those that are marketed under the name of colon cleansers. Colon cleansing is essential if you want to lose weight fast as it will eliminate any waste that is left in your intestines. This can help you lose weight at a dramatic speed if you use it often.

It is important that you drink plenty of water when you are body detoxification to lose weight. You never want to go on diet without supplementing yourself with water. By drinking 8 glasses of water a day and using a good, natural body detoxifier, you will take off weight quicker than dieting alone.

Of course, it goes without saying that you should exercise good common sense when you are trying to lose weight with body detoxification. Body detoxification is not a magic formula that lets you just lose weight while eating what you want. You still need to increase your activity as well as reduce the amount of calories that you are consuming. Body detoxification will, however, be an asset to your weight loss and will enable you to take in nutrients while cleansing your body of waste, helping you to lose weight.

Importance in Choosing the Right Product

When you are looking for body detoxification products, you have quite a choice. You can go online to look for products or purchase them from health food stores or suppliers. One thing that you will want to be certain of is that the body detoxification products are made from natural products.

You can choose the following when you are home body detoxification:

- Pre-made formulas
- Tablets
- Powders for mixing with water
- Teas
- Patches
- Aromatherapy
- Foot therapy

Many people choose more than one product for home body detoxification. All work differently but achieve the same results.

Here is a rundown of each of the products and how they can work to cleanse your body:

Pre-made formulas

Of all of the body detoxification products, pre-made formulas are the most costly. This is because all of the work has been done and the formula is ready to use as is. Those who are looking for convenience are better off to use pre-made formulas for body detoxification.

You can purchase these formulas in many different outlets. These include high end salons, health food stores and online outlets. Using the pre-made formulas is easy enough to do. Simply follow the instructions on the label and you will accomplish the cleansing at home. You can find body detoxification solutions in a variety of different flavors. Most of them are loaded with vitamins and juices, such as Acai berry, a noted and powerful antioxidant. Pre-made formulas are ideal for anyone who does not have the time or the inclination to make their own formula. They can be used with other methods of body detoxification to get a true body cleanse.

Tablets

There are hundreds of different tablets that are made for body detoxification. The tablets work less quickly than the solutions, although they are very effective. Many people take the tablets on a daily basis to keep their body cleansed.

Most of the tablets that are used for body detoxification are made from derivatives of herbs as well as vitamins. Some fruits, like the Acai Berry, often used in body detoxification, are only available in juice or powder form in most areas of the world. Tablets usually contain components like Acai, the antioxidant, as well as cranberry, lemon and other ingredients that are known to flush out the system effectively. Those who want a product that will work over a period of time will enjoy using the body detoxification tablets that are on the market. You can purchase these tablets at health food stores, online outlets and even the local drugstore. Make sure that the body detoxification tablets that you purchase are all natural and contain all natural ingredients. You can even find that there are some organic tablets that are sold by distributors.

Powders for Mixing

If you like the fast action of the body detoxification solutions but do not want to pay the price, you can create your own body detoxification solution with powders that you purchase at a variety of different places, including online. You simply have to mix the powder with purified water and you are all set to drink. You will find the powders in a variety of different flavors and can even get them in a variety pack so that you can sample several different flavors to see which ones you like.

You use powders for mixing in the same manner as you would use a pre-made solution. Follow the directions on the label as different products have different directions. The pre-made powders are ideal for anyone who wants to save money but likes the idea of using a body detoxification formula that they can drink.

Teas

Drinking green tea is very good for body detoxification but drinking green tea that is fortified with more antioxidants and vitamins is even better for your body. You can make the tea as you would a normal cup of brewed tea and take it either hot or cold. Again, you will want to follow the directions on the package when you are using teas as a way to cleanse your body.

Teas are ideal for those who like to drink tea and are looking for a soothing way to naturally cleanse their body at home. They work quickly but not as quickly as the solutions. Like the tablets, the teas are often used for a long term cleansing basis.

Patches

Just like you can get a nicotine patch to help you quit smoking, you can also use a patch to cleanse your body. A patch for body detoxification is used the same way. You put the patch on your skin and the properties are absorbed into your bloodstream through your skin. This is a slower way to cleanse your body, but may be more convenient for those who are busy and do not have time to spend with a solution.

You can purchase the body detoxification patches at a number of different outlets. All of the same outlets that sell body detoxification supplies usually sell patches. If you are the type of person who does not have a lot of time to spend on body detoxification and does not want to drink teas or solutions, the patch is ideal for you. You just have to put it on and you are all set.

Aromatherapy

One way that you can naturally cleanse your body is through aromatherapy. Aromatherapy can be used in two different ways. You can put essential oils on the skin and also breathe them in. Some essential oils such as those derived from lemon and tea tree leaves work well to cleanse the body.

You should not put essential oil directly on your skin as it can be very potent. You should mix essential oils with carrier oil such as canola oil, and then massage into the skin. The skin absorbs the essential oils in the same manner as the patch and it goes into the bloodstream.

You can also use aromatherapy to inhale the essential oils into the lungs so that they are also transported into the bloodstream in this manner. You need to use an infuser to inhale the oils.

Aromatherapy is good for body detoxification on a long term basis. It does not work quickly, but is effective. It is similar to the patches in that it is absorbed into the bloodstream and works to cleanse all parts of the body, including the digestive system. They work well for those who want to have a long term body detoxification experience at home.

Foot Therapy

Your feet are the pathway to your body and foot therapy can work well to cleanse your body from impurities. Foot therapy usually consists of massage or magnetic therapy. Both can work well for body detoxification and work on the long term basis. You can use homemade remedies when you practice foot therapy at home.

Foot therapy is often used in conjunction with other body detoxification methods as a way to not only cleanse the body but also to keep it clean and healthy.

Chapter 5- How Does Detoxification Help in Losing Weight?

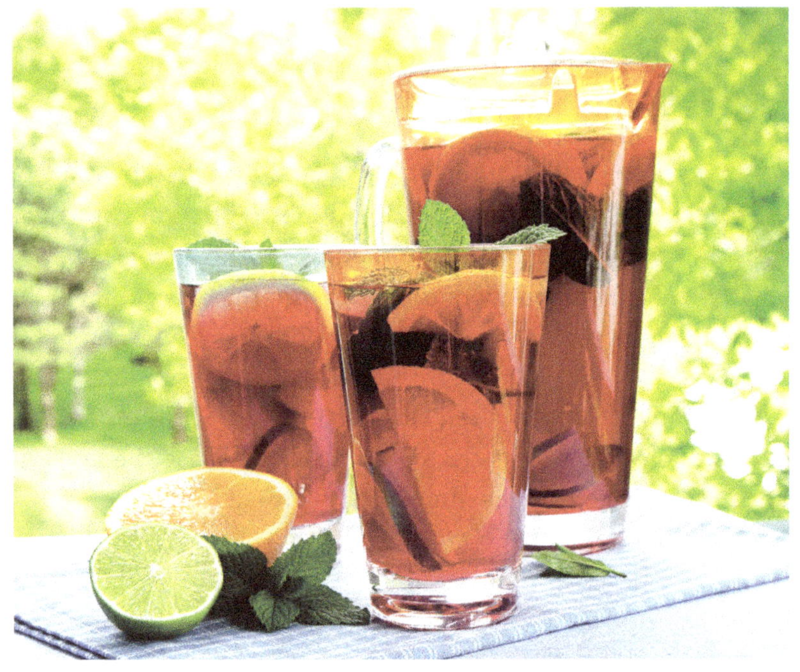

One of the main reasons why you should look to detoxify your body is for weight loss. In fact, because weight loss is such a good side benefit of detoxification there have been a lot of products and diets to come out recently that claim they will help you with detoxification and weight loss.

The detoxification process seems like a complete contradiction to the way people normally lose weight and get healthy. Unlike diets where you count calories, a detoxification plan encourages you to eat certain foods that will help your body gently get rid of toxins and other problematic elements in your system. As you change your diet to include these new foods, your body will begin to get rid of what doesn't serve it anymore.

Depending on your lifestyle, there may be just a few things causing problems in your system or there could be a large amount of "junk" clogging up your body's normal processes. Here are some of the elements that can be eliminated from you body through detoxification:

- Artificial sweeteners
- Pesticides
- Preservatives
- Artificial colors

These elements can cause you to gain weight because they inhibit your liver. It's primarily your liver's job to filter out harmful chemicals in your body. If you are bombarding your system with harmful chemicals each day, your liver gets overtaxed and doesn't work as efficiently.

If this were any other organ this wouldn't make you cause weight, but your liver is also responsible for metabolizing fat. If your liver is overtaxed from the large amount of chemicals and non-foods that you are eating, your body will store fat more quickly. Your body will also be unable to use the excess fat that you store as energy. As a result, you'll not only gain weight but be unable to shed your weight effectively.

When you understand this process, it's easy to see why a toxic diet can cause weight gain. When you take the time to detoxify your body, your organs will be able to efficiently use the energy that you eat during your meals. You'll naturally start to lose weight because your liver will be processing your food correctly and not storing all of the calories as fat.

However, the key is in finding the right type of detoxification method that will work for you and keep your body healthy.

Detox Diet and Its Magic

Since detoxification can help your weight loss efforts, it's only natural that lots of manufacturers are out there claiming that specific Detox diets are what you need to restore your good health. If you've spent any amount of time researching detoxification, you've probably been overwhelmed with information about detoxification diets. You may be wondering if they are worth your time and money.

There are tons of products online and in health food stores that promise that you'll receive detoxification benefits by taking pills, powders or other supplements. You can save your money and leave these products on the shelves.

It's not that detoxifying the body is a bad idea; it's just that you don't need to pay through the nose or starve yourself in order to have detoxification effects. Later on in this report you'll learn some simple techniques for detoxifying your system safely and effectively.

Overall, health experts agree that eating better and drinking more water is all that you need in order to detoxify your body. The concept that you need to take fancy pills or powders in order to Detox is nothing more than an empty promise by manufacturers that want to make money off of your fears.

Here are some common Detox diet scams that you should avoid:

- The Master Cleanse Detox diet (starving yourself for five to ten days with a variation of lemonade)
- Carbohydrate blocking pills
- -The Fruit Flush plan (eating nothing more than fruit and protein drinks)
- -Colon cleansing pills -Intestinal drawing formula

There are tons of other plans and products that claim that they will help Detox your body. Later in this report, you'll learn the truth about detoxification. It's a lot simpler than money hungry manufacturers would have you think.

Do Detox Foot Pad Effective

Second to detoxification diets, Detox foot pads are one of the most popular detoxification products promoted by unscrupulous manufacturers. These have been heavily marketed online and on television. According to manufacturers, foot pads will draw out the toxins from the bottom of your feet.

When you place the pads on your feet at night, special ingredients in the pad can draw out toxins and other harmful elements from the body...or at least that's what manufacturers claim!

The foot pads work using the principles of reflexology. According to reflexology, there are points on the bottom of your feet that correspond to all of your major body systems. When you treat the bottom of your feet, you can supposedly treat the rest of your body as well. The pads cover the soles of the feet and cover the portions of the foot that correspond to major bodily systems.

Detox Cleanse Made Easy

The first flaw in the logic behind a foot pad Detox is the role of our skin in detoxifying the body. Although some nutrients pass back and forth through the skin, heavy metal deposits and other toxins cannot get into the body through skin. If they can't get in, there's no way that they are going to be able to get out by simply wearing pads on your foot at night.

The second flaw is in their design. If you've seen the commercials for foot Detox pads or watched videos of the Detox pads, you'll notice that after using the pads the surface of the pads turn dark. This is supposed to be an indicator that they are working to remove toxins from the body.

Most are made from Tourmaline, which is a stone that produces negative ions and bamboo vinegar which is supposedly going to help your body eliminate toxins through the skin.

The color change that is seen after wearing the patches is a result of the ingredients themselves. The bamboo vinegar is dried and placed into the foot pad along with all of the other ingredients. When the bamboo vinegar is exposed to moisture, like the sweat from your feet at night, it returns back to its liquid form.

When your feet sweat at night, the vinegar changes colors and as a result, the pads appear dark when you take them off in the morning.

However, if you haven't done the research it might seem like the foot pads are doing their job. To help educate you on the true nature of this product, here are three case studies of the most popular types of foot pads that are available.

Case Study #1: Kinoki Detox Foot Pads

These foot pads have been heavily advertised on television and online heavily. In the past several months Kinoki foot pads have been the object of media scrutiny and online discussion. They were even featured on an episode of the American television show "20/20."

How it Works

The manufacturer of Kinoki foot pads claim that they work by pulling toxins and other harmful ingredients out of your body through your feet. According to their marketing materials, the pads use "Ions" in order to make your body healthy.

At nighttime, users are supposed to place the pads on each of their feet. They should rest for 8 to 10 hours for best results. In the morning, the foot pads will be removed. Users are supposed to use them for at least a week in order to completely remove toxins from their body. In addition to removing toxins, Kinoki foot pads are supposed to also remove parasites, mucous, chemicals and cellulite.

There are several ingredients in the Kinoki foot pad that are supposed to be good for detoxifying your body. The ingredients included are bamboo vinegar, chitin, tourmaline and assorted Chinese herbs. These ingredients have not been scientifically proven to have any benefit when it comes to detoxification.

Do Kinoki Foot Pads Work?

At the time of this writing, the official website of the Kinoki food pads has been taken off the web if that gives you any indication of their effectiveness. If you search online for reviews, you'll find scores of people who were ripped off by this company and who wasted their money on a product that does not work.

In the "20/20" report, they were exposed to be a scam with clinical tests that showed that there were no heavy metals or toxins in the pads after wearing them. The pads basically amount to an expensive vinegar patches.

Case Study #2: Dr. Group's Detox Foot Pads

Dr. Group' Detox Foot Pads may be less well known than Kinoki food pads but they operate by much of the same principles. The manufacturers claim that when you use Dr. Group's Detox foot pads they will remove harmful chemicals and heavy metals from your system.

How it Works

Dr. Group's foot pads differ from other foot pads in that they use organic ingredients. According to their website, they are the world's only Detox pads that are designed for chemical, toxin and heavy metal ions.

Like other Detox pads, Dr. Group's pads claim to use reflexology points to draw out toxins from your system. The pads stimulate the surface of the bottom of your skin to release toxins. In addition to wearing the foot pads, you can also increase your detoxification benefits from the pads by stimulating acupressure points on the bottom of your feet before applying the pads.

To use the pads, you need to remove the backing sheet from the pad. Apply the pads to the bottom of both feet just before going to bed. Leave the foot pads on while you sleep (preferably for 8 to 10 hours). In the morning, you'll see that the pads have turned darker.

According to the manufacturer, the more you use the pad, the lighter they will be in the morning. This is evidence of the pads taking toxins out of your body.

You should use the pads once per week for the whole night. Make sure to drink lots of purified water throughout the day to help your body eliminate toxins. The pads may need to be worn for up to 12 months depending on the level of toxins in your body.

Does It Work?

Although there certainly is a lot less bad press about Dr. Group's foot patches than Kinoki foot pads, the results aren't exactly outstanding. Although some people claim that they do see results after continued use, there is no scientific evidence that they are actually eliminating toxins from their body. At $35.95 for a five night supply, it will cost you a bit to test these pads out for yourself.

Case Study #3: Cleanse Patch

How it Works

Like the other types of Detox foot pads, Cleanse Patches promise to remove heavy metals and toxins from your body when you wear them on your feet at night. According to the product description, you are supposed to wear the pads each night for five days in a row.

The active ingredients in Cleanse Patches are organic Agaricus mushroom, organic tourmaline and organic eucalyptus sap powder. These ingredients combine together without fillers in order to have a deep cleansing experience, according to the product's website.

Does It Work?

Although the manufacturers of cleanse patches claim that only their product has this unique blend of Detox ingredients, these patches offer no better results than any other foot patches on the market. The claims made on the product's website are quickly refuted by learning about the science of detoxification and the truth about how the detoxification works.

Detox Diet and Detox Foot Patches Needed?

Now that you know some of the facts about Detox diets and foot pads you probably realize that you don't need these products in order to detoxify your system. These products are completely unnecessary. They are a waste of your money and in some cases, can actually be harmful to your health.

A lot of the reasons that people use detoxification products simply can't be achieved. Many people think that weight loss is a natural result of detoxification. While you can lose some weight while on a detoxification diet, you will likely gain the weight back once you go to your normal form of eating.

They think that detoxifying their body would help kick start their weight loss, but in reality it creates poor eating habits and sets you up for a metabolic roller coaster. Unless you make lasting changes in your body, you won't keep the weight off. Another main reason people seek out detoxification is to clean out the digestive system.

According to the proponents of detoxification, you need special pills, powders or foot pads to rid your gut of old food particles, parasites and toxins. These effects can be achieved by eating more fiber and drinking more water.

You don't need to buy expensive products and you don't need to use harsh methods to detoxify your system.

Chapter 6- Recipes for Home-made Detox Drinks

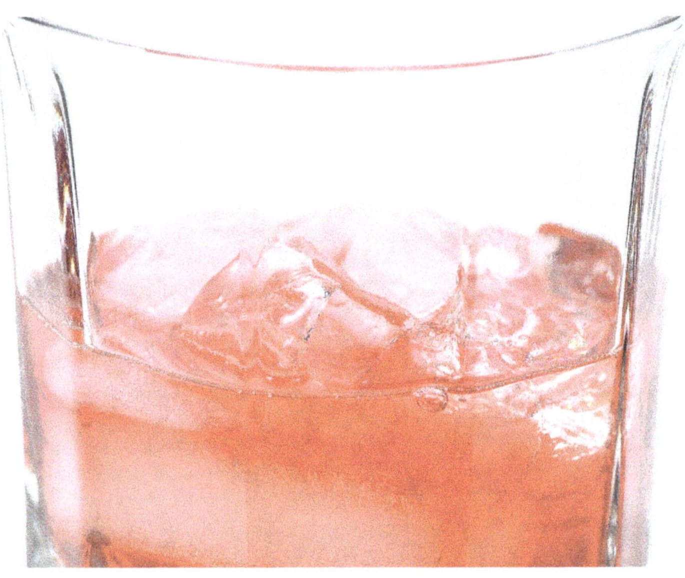

You can easily make your own home made remedies that are ideal for home body detoxification. This chapter will explore the different remedies that you can use and where you can get the ingredients for these body detoxification solutions.

For all of these homemade remedies, use only purified water. You can purchase purified water in the grocery store or get it right out of your tap if you have a water purifying system in your home. If you do not have a water purifying system, you should consider getting one for your home. This can help you keep your body free from some of the impurities you get from water.

Body Detoxifier One - Lemon Pepper Cleanser

Both lemon and pepper combined will work well to zip through the body as a cleanser. Lemon pepper cleanser is one of the easiest and effective home cleansing remedies.

8 Ounces of Water

2 Teaspoons of lemon zest

½ Teaspoon of black pepper

Combine the water and the other ingredients and drink it down. After you are finished drinking the solution, drink two 8 ounce glasses of water. This will help flush the solution into your system. Lemon pepper cleanser is good for the colon and entire digestive system.

For best results, use fresh ground black pepper and fresh lemon zest from a fresh lemon.

Alternate use - You can omit the black pepper and add one teaspoon of fresh lemon juice to the mix

Body Detoxifier Two - Italian body detoxifier

8 Ounces of Water

1 Teaspoon of flax seed oil

1 Teaspoon of Basil

1 Teaspoon of Oregano

½ Teaspoon of Garlic

Combine all of the ingredients with the water and drink it. After drinking, wait five minutes for the solution to settle and then drink two more glasses of water. This acts as a detoxifier for the entire body and is good for both the digestive system as well as the circulatory system.

For best results, use fresh herbs and garlic.

Alternate use - You can substitute Rosemary for Basil.

Body Detoxifier Three - Berry Detox

6 Ounces of Water

2 Ounces of Pure Acai Berry Juice

½ Cup Blueberries

4 Fresh Strawberries

Put all of the ingredients in the blender and mix them together. Drink them and follow the solution with an 8 ounce glass of purified water. This is a detoxifier that is loaded with antioxidants and purifiers.

For best results, use only fresh ingredients.

Alternate use - Substitute ½ cup of blueberries for the strawberries.

Body Detoxifier Four - Tropical Detox

1 Banana

1 cup unsweetened, plain yogurt

½ cup pure orange juice

½ cup pure pineapple juice

Put all ingredients into a blender and the mix them. This will be more like a shake than a traditional drink but works well to cleanse out the digestive tract as well as provide essential nutrients. This works slower than other body detoxifiers but is healthy for the colon as well as the heart and immune system.

For best results - Use only fresh ingredients and pure juices

Alternative - You can 1 cup of orange juice instead of half and half of pineapple juice and orange juice.

Body Detoxifier Five - Energizing Cleanse

8 Ounces of Water

1 Teaspoon of Maca Root

1 Teaspoon of Ginseng

1 Teaspoon of Acai powder

You may have to use pestle and mortar to break up the roots, especially if they are fresh, as they should be. You can purchase liquid Ginseng, although you are better off to purchase capsule forms. Grind up the dry ingredients, mix them with the Acai powder and then add them to the water. Drink down the mixture and then drink another glass of water.

This will not only give you energy to spare, but will also work towards detoxifying your digestive and circulatory system. If you are looking for a way to energize your body, this will do it.

You can purchase the supplements in any health food store or even online. Make sure that they are pure supplements and not just chemically reproduced. Ginseng is often available in "energy drinks" in stores - avoid that and get the actual product.

Body Detoxifier Six - Colon Cleanse Diet

8 Ounces of Water

1 Teaspoon of Flax Seed Oil

1 Teaspoon of FRESH ginger

1 Teaspoon of Grape seed oil

1 Package of green tea

This is a body detoxifier that works well as a colon cleanser. Add the ingredients together before adding to the water. You may need to use the mortar and pestle to grind up the ginger if you do not have a food processor. You want only to use fresh ginger for this cleanse. Open up the package of green tea and dump it into the mix.

Mix everything with the water and then drink. Follow it with two glasses of water. This is a good weight loss detoxifier that you can make right from products that you purchase at the supermarket.

For best results, Use only fresh ingredients that are pure

Alternate use - Use a green tea capsule and grind it up with the mortar and pestle.

Body Detoxifier Seven - Cinnamon Spice

1 cup of brewed green tea

1 teaspoon of honey

½ teaspoon of cinnamon

After you have brewed the green tea, add the cinnamon and the honey to the mixture and drink it hot. This is a pleasant tasting drink and will not only relax you, but will also cleanse out your body and help your heart.

For best results - Use fresh ground cinnamon

Body Detoxifier Eight - Kidney Cleansing

8 Ounces of Water

½ Cup pure cranberry juice

¼ Cup pure Acai juice

3 Teaspoons orange juice

Mix the ingredients together and add them to the water. Drink it down and then drink two more 8 ounce glasses of water. This will help clean out your urinary tract and clear up urinary tract infections.

For best results - Use only pure ingredients and 100 percent pure orange juice

Body Detoxifier Nine - Lavender Cleansing

8 Ounces of Water

1 Teaspoon of pure Lavender oil

1 Teaspoon of Flax Seed oil

Mix the oils with the water and drink. Consume another glass of water after to flush down the mixture. This is a total body cleanse and will detoxify all parts of your body.

Warning - Use only pure Lavender oil. Essential oils, with the exception of a few, are not made for ingestion Lavender oil is an exception, but it must be pure.

Body Detoxifier Ten - Tropical Delight

Ice Cubes made from purified water

½ Banana

1 Teaspoon of Flax Seed Oil

½ Cup orange juice

¼ Cup Acai juice

2 Teaspoons of Lemon juice (pure)

Mix all of the ingredients together in a blender. Add enough ice cubes to fill the blender and then purifier. Drink the entire amount of the potion. This is a detoxifier for the body and can also substitute as a meal if you are trying to lose weight.

Body Detoxifier Eleven - Veggie Cleanser

1 Fresh Carrot, peeled

2 Crowns of Broccoli

1 Teaspoon of Omega Fish Oil

1 Teaspoon Flax Seed Oil

Ice Cubes

You need a food processor for this recipe, although it certainly cleans out the system and works wonders on the digestive system. You have to pulverize the vegetables so that they are like mush and then add the ice cubes and oils to the mix. Mix well and then consume the entire amount. Follow with a glass of purified water.

This is a safe and healthy drink that can be consumed on a healthy basis. It can also be used as a substitute for a meal if you are dieting.

Body Detoxifier Twelve - Vitamin Cleanser

1 Cup Green Tea - Hot

1 Capsule of Vitamin D

1 Capsule of Vitamin A

1 Capsule of Vitamin K

½ Teaspoon of Cinnamon

Grind up the capsules in a mortar and then add them to the hot tea so that they dissolve. Then add the cinnamon to the mix. Drink it down. This will add vitamins and nutrients to your body that you may be lacking. It is good for eliminating stress, depression and also healthy for the heart.

All of the ingredients for these body detoxifiers can be found at your local grocery store or health food store. You need to make sure that you are purchasing pure ingredients and not those made from synthetics. You can buy a mortar and pestle online or in some drugstores and health food stores.

Home-made Remedies for Skin

Drinking solutions is one of the best ways to detoxify the body but not the only way. There are many who do not want to take the solutions for a variety of different reasons, or who also want additional body detoxification.

Using massage oils made from essential oils is one way that you can work to detoxify your body on a long term scale. Essential oils should never be used directly on the skin, with the exception of Rose and Lavender, as they can cause a reaction. As discussed earlier, aromatherapy works to detoxify your body in a slower way and will work continually over a period of time.

You can find essential oils for these recipes online or in some health food stores. It is very important that you use pure essential oils or extracts for these recipes as synthetics will not give you the same results. These recipes are all safe to use topically as massage oils. You can also use the alternate recipes, given after the massage

These are all safe and tested recipes for aromatherapy style detoxification:

Aromatherapy Body Detoxification One - Lavender and Rose

This is one of the easiest of all of the aromatherapy detoxification recipes. It combines two of the safest essential oils that will not only relax you, but cleanse your body of its impurities.

½ Cup Lavender Oil

¼ Cup Rose Oil

Mix well together and then massage onto your feet, neck and chest area. The essential oils will be absorbed into your skin and then into your blood stream. This is a good recipe for those who are tense and want to relax, while detoxifying their body at the same time.

You can also put the oils directly into an infuser and breath in the scent. This will allow it to be absorbed into the lungs.

Another alternate to this recipe is to put the oils in your bath and soak in them. You will start to feel relaxed right away as you will not only be breathing in the oils, but allowing them to soak into your bloodstream through your skin.

Remember, lavender and rose are the only essential oils that are safe to put directly on the skin. The rest of the recipes will involve the use of carrier oil for direct skin contact.

Aromatherapy Body Detoxification Two - Frankincense

Frankincense has been used as a healing potent for thousands of years. You can use this as a way to get rid of body toxins as well as help your circulatory system:

1 Cup Carrier Oil (such as canola oil)

1 Teaspoon of pure Frankincense

Mix the oils together well. You should put them in a dark bottle with a cork lid for the best results. Once they are mixed together, you can then use them as massage oil. Rub the soles of your feet with this mixture as well as the chest area. This will do wonders for your circulatory system and the scent is pleasant. If you have a partner, see if they will massage your back.

You can get canola oil at any grocery store. Frankincense is a common essential oil that can be used as a body detoxifier and is found at most health food stores. Remember to only use pure Frankincense for this recipe.

You can also put the oil in an infuser and breathe in. Because the scent of this essential oil is so pleasant, many people choose to not only use it as a massage oil, but also as a relaxing scent.

Aromatherapy Body Detoxification Three - Tea Tree Oil & Lemon

Both Tree Tea Oil and Lemon Oil are useful when it come to helping the digestive system. If you want to lose weight as well as clear out your digestive system so that it works well, you can make this mix at home and use it as massage oil or in an infuser:

1 Cup Carrier Oil (such as canola oil)

½ Teaspoon of Tea Tree Oil

½ Teaspoon of Pure lemon oil (not lemon juice)

Mix the oils together in a brown bottle and shake. Use them in the same manner as you use the other aromatherapy massage oils. You can also inhale them in the infuser.

Be sure to get pure lemon oil and not lemon juice. Pure lemon extract will work as a substitute for this type of detoxification if you cannot find pure lemon oil. Tea Tree oil is available at most health food stores - just be sure that it is pure and not made from synthetics.

Aromatherapy Body Detoxification Four - Almond

This is one of the aromatherapy treatments that you can use from extracts that are readily available in the grocery store. You should still use a carrier oil when you are using extracts.

1 Cup Carrier oil (such as canola oil)

1 Teaspoon of pure Almond Extract

1 Teaspoon of pure Vanilla Extract

Combine all of the products and shake well in the bottle. You can then apply on the skin. The scent is very nice and you can also burn the oils on their own by their infuser. This is a body detoxification that will work to bolster the immune system and clear out any toxins. Best of all, you can easily find the extracts when you are in the store.

Using massage therapy and breathing in the essential oils is one way that you can detoxify your body at home. In addition to using these techniques, however you should still practice good habits such as not smoking, limiting your alcohol intake and drinking plenty of water.

Stay Detoxified

Home body detoxification is not difficult and there are many choices from which to choose when it comes to what type of remedy you want to use. You may want to start slow when it comes to trying to detoxify your body and drink the detox teas.

If you go online, you will see a myriad of many detoxification kits, teas, pills, drinks and just about anything else. While these work to help you detoxify your body, it is very important that you understand that they are not a magic cure. In other words, you cannot expect to party all of the time, abuse your body and then cure it by using detox.

Home detoxification can, however, rid your body of toxins and get you clean. If you have been abusing tobacco, alcohol or drugs, you can clean up your act at home and use the body detoxification formulas mentioned here to get your body clean.

Before using a body detoxification system, you should use a colon cleanser. This will help you clear out your colon and will allow it to be more receptive to the vitamins and nutrients that you are providing your body. A healthy digestive tract is the start of a healthy body.

To stay detoxified, use an at home body detoxification system once every week and eat a healthy diet loaded with vitamins and minerals. Drink plenty of water a day and exercise. Take a multi vitamin and a supplement of vitamin C.

You can get your body into shape by using home detoxification methods that are mentioned in this book as well as those that you purchase in the store. You just have to be persistent with the methods. If you fall back and revert to an unhealthy habit, look at it as a setback but not the end of the world.

Detoxify and then start over again to try to maintain good health for your entire body by ridding yourself of toxins.

CHAPTER 7- ADDICTION AND THE ROLE OF DETOXIFICATION

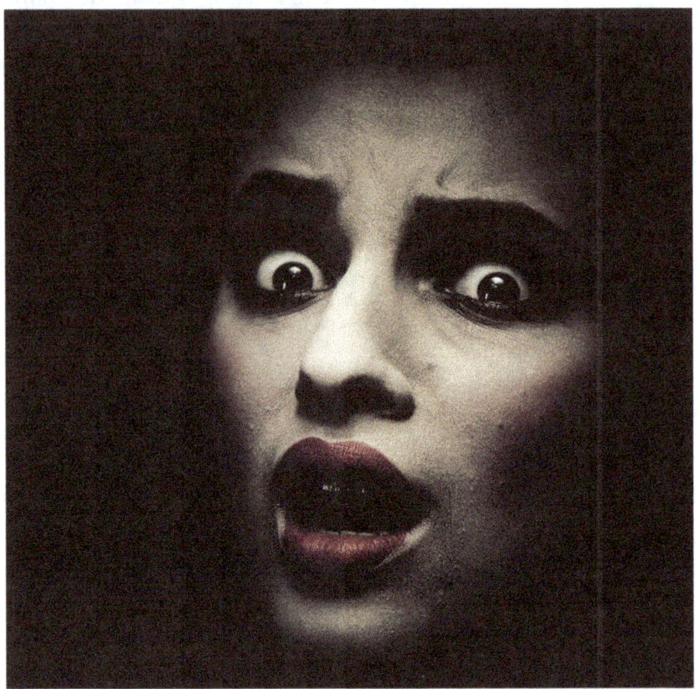

Food addictions

Lots of individuals struggle with this type of addition and it is usually directed at the draw to sweetened and overly salted food types. Both these groups are bad for health and if there is the added factor of fatty foods thrown into the combination, then the effects can be detrimental indeed.

Most of this type of addiction has been found to be linked to the psychological disposition of the individual, therefore treating this aspect in the overall exercise to overcome the addiction is very important to the eventual desired success.

Intravenous amino acids addictions

Here the detoxification method used includes amino acid therapy where the physical work out, infra red sauna; acupuncture and massage are all complimenting elements to the specific nutritional plan laid out to combat this addiction.

The use of herbs and natural nutritious foods will eventually help to restore the chemical imbalance in the body system which is causing the individual's health to deteriorate due to the substance abuse.

A careful selection of nutrition supplements, vitamins and herbs can help in the addiction kicking exercise. Besides slowly restoring the balance within the body system, these inclusions in the daily diet plan can also help to eliminate simple starches and sugars from the system. Good nutrition can also help the addict and heal the damage done to the body due to the substance abuse.

Relationship between Nutrition and Addiction

Most addictions cause the individual to have poor health due to the abuse the body goes through because of the addiction to the specific negative elements.

Therefore taking the first step towards improving the health conditions of the patient would be something to consider. This is more likely to make a positive impact on the individual undergoing the nutritional treatment as the general health conditions can certainly be seen to improve dramatically.

Improved health conditions will then give the addict the energy and zest to keep up with the rehabilitation program thus allowing a comfortable time frame for the desired results to be achieved.

The biochemistry in the brain of an addict has been altered drastically through the abuse of such negative substances, and the recovery time the brain needs, will be further shortened if there is a good nutritional plan in place to speed this along effectively. Other areas that would need attention would in the high levels of trans fatty acids found in a lot of foods consumed thus the need for a healthy, balanced meal program that is nutritionally adequate to combat the preceding negative condition.

Combining this nutritionally balanced diet plan with a proper exercise regimen, the brain conditions will be able to be more receptive to other changes that are being attempted towards the recovery state of the individual.

There has been a lot of proven scientific research that supports the positive effects good nutrition can have in treating certain addictions. The success rates are based on the individual's focus on the nutritional value of the whole exercise.

Chapter 8- Detoxification and Choosing the Right Nutrition to Beat Addiction

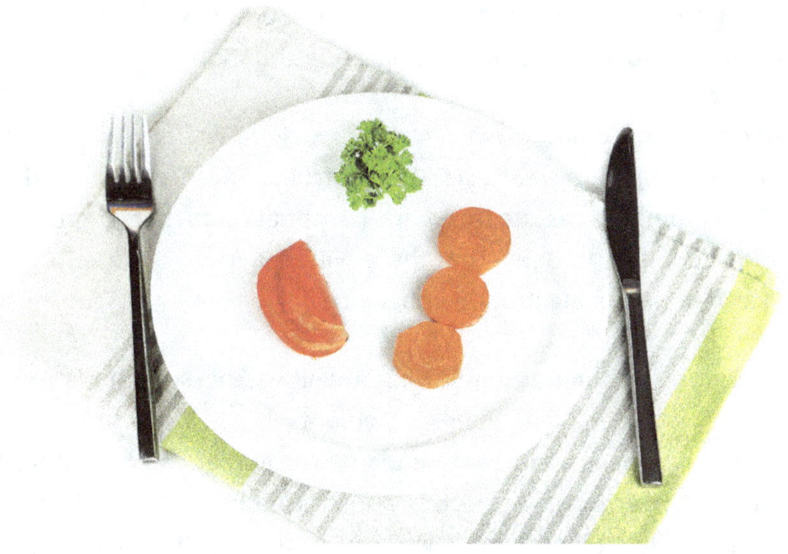

Almost all addictions in some ways cause gradual and progressive damage to the various parts of the human body.

These may include damage to the brain, organs, hormones, immune and nervous systems, but the good news is that by treating these with good nutrition can eventually bring the addict back to a healthy body and mind condition.

Alcohol, drugs and junk foods are the most common addictions that most people struggle to kick. This affects the complexity of the body system in a negative way and usually causes the sufferer to fall further away from any chance of recovery. Therefore treating the deteriorating body condition with a healthy and nutritional diet plan would be one way of bringing the individual back to some semblance of good health.

Alcohol is a major addiction problem that causes the nutritional deficiency in the addict. The liver detoxifies harmful substances and the pancreas regulated the bold sugar and absorption of fats into the system and when there is alcohol abuse these body parts and their contributing mechanisms are severely compromised. Counter acting this with a good dose of vitamin B6, thiamine and folic acid could help to improve the deteriorating situation.

Addiction of opiates which would include codeine heroin and morphine generally affects the gastrointestinal system and this very commonly results in severe constipation. When treating this addiction, it is probable that there will be a loss of nutrients which is evident in the electrolyte imbalances.

Therefore creating and following a well balances meal plan which would include high fiber ingredients such as whole grains, vegetables, peas and beans would be recommended to restore the balance. Liver disease which is also caused by addiction to certain negative substances will also cause the health problems but including the appropriate doses of vitamin A and E into the diet plan would help tremendously.

Detox for Addicts

The introduction of negative substances into the body's system will definitely cause a lot of damage, in the long run both to the mental and physical state. However all is not lost, as there are many possibilities available to try and treat this negative condition once the individual is willing to acknowledge and work towards a positive turn around.

Detoxification for addiction is just one if the more popular recourses used of late. Incorporating nutritional elements into the detoxification exercise will help the addict build up a healthy body condition which will help to further strengthen the resolve to beat the negative addiction.

When the individual is in better health, the chances of being able to have the necessary positive mind set and positive body conditions will be evident, thus effectively creating less stress on the individual at a time when all seems against him or her.

The immune status and general health can be improved greatly through the use of a proper nutritional diet plan.

Some scientific research conducted have been able to show conclusively, that the inclusion of a well balanced and nutritional diet plan can be pivotal in the recovery period of the addict.

The inclusion of nutrients such as minerals, vitamins B6, magnesium, folate and vitamin E, have all shown to dramatically and positively impact the detoxification exercise.

This significant change for the better is very encouraging to those intending to attempt the detoxification program especially if it is for the first time.

This natural use of nutrients to launch the detoxification exercise will help the individual come out of the experience in better health both mentally and physically.

However it should be noted that all detoxification exercises should be done with the appropriate amount of knowledge on the use of the various natural remedies and with some supervision.

CHAPTER 9- DETOXIFYING ADDICTION AWAY

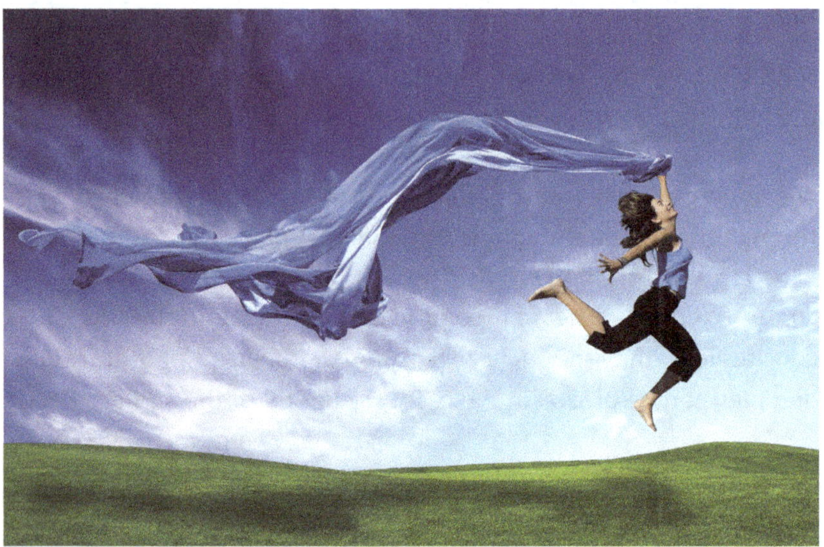

Seeking alternative that are less stressful and painful are usually the more popular choices made when it comes to trying to beat an addiction. These addictions may not necessary only be linked to the society shunning kind, and generally cover almost anything and everything and is commonly recognized in the individual's inability to turn away from something comfortably.

Juicing has been documented as being a very helpful way of beating an addiction. Most practitioners believe that blended and juiced ingredients can contribute to the first steps towards healing both the body and mind, as it provides the body with the ideal conditions for energized output. Juicing is a very quick and easy way to put the balance back into the cells in the body system so that the process of rejuvenation can take place effectively and according to the needs of the individual.

Juicing has been documented to address issues such as elevating energy levels to the requirements of the individual, changing the molecular conditions by providing the essential chemical balance needed, keeping the mental faculties healthy and not focused on the need to have instant relief for anything and many other positive contributions.

When it comes to cleaning the molecular conditions to ensure optimum productivity the use of juicing for "green drinks" concoctions is most beneficial. The wealth of antioxidants, saponins, polyphenols, proanthrocyanidins, bioflavonoid and may other positive elements all be found in the juices that are designed to provide such nourishments.

All these elements are needed by the body system to enhance the cleansing, healing and rejuvenation of the various parts that contribute to the overall ideal health conditions of the individual indulging in the juicing exercise. To kick the addiction habit, the addict will need all the outside help for the body to be able to cope with the sudden deprivation of the negative substances used throughout the addiction phase.

Vitamins for Addicts

In the quest to regain the ideal health conditions enjoyed before the onset of the addiction, the individual would be well advised to seek recommendations on a good vitamin regimen that will promote and rejuvenate the body systems so that optimal health is evident.

Through the course on the addiction indulgence, it is very likely that the body has sustained significant damage and getting it back to its optimum state, will require all the outside help it can get.

This uphill battle can be assisted and eased somewhat with the inclusion of proper vitamins designed to focus on specific areas that need immediate attention.

There are several different supplements that can be used to aid in the process to bring the addicts health back to its optimum and these may include taking vitamins with zinc and vitamin C content. Antioxidants that have the ability to neutralize free radical would come from sources such as beta-carotene, vitamins C and E, zinc and selenium.

There is also the advantage of taking vitamin B and particularly vitamin B1. Supplements with calcium and magnesium are also recommended, while the use of B complex, chromium and vitamin C are also becoming popular nutritional therapy ingredients.

Vitamins such vitamin B complex 50, Pantothenic acid Niacin, Calcium, Magnesium, Amino Acid Mix, L-Glutamine, L- Tyrosine are all good elements to include when designing a nutritional plan to combat the drug addiction condition in an effective and natural way.

Using essential fatty acids which would come from the flaxseed can also be helpful in the treatment of drug addiction. Other vitamins that could be useful in fighting addition would be niacin and calcium which are needed and instrumental in maintaining proper brain functions. The energy source provided by the L-Phenylalanine is also another important nutritional ingredient that is needed for optimum brain functions.

Massage Therapy

In the quest to overcome any sort of addiction, there is a need to explore as many options as possible and then identify the ones most useful and beneficial in managing to produce the desired results.

Massage therapy is something that has found a place in the struggle towards beating the addiction, as it is able to provide the mental and physical therapeutic experience that is both calming and effective.

Addiction or substance abuse usually causes major health problems for those in this predicament and also for those linked to the addict. Incorporating massage into the program will allow the addict to have some level of relief at all the various stages of the withdrawal phase and this would include the quitting stage, the withdrawal stage, the detoxification stage and the eventual abstinence stage.

The physical, emotional and spiritual phase of the recovery period can directly benefit from the therapeutic touch that is the product of the massage sessions.

As the skin is the largest sensory organ of the human body, attention given to the aspect especially if the attention is of the positive kind, the ensuing results will definitely be positive.

Massage therapy is ideally designed to address and benefit in areas that might not be as effectively or as quickly affected through the other treatment methods.

With the use of massage, the addiction treatment will allow for the release of the neurotransmitter dopamine which is actually the chemical messenger responsible for making the body and mind be encompassed with the feel good aura. This is definitely a good frame of body and mind to be in especially when the usual withdrawal phase can be painful and rather challenging to face. This then helps to keep the individual focused on gaining back the original mental and physical idealness evident, before the onset of the addiction.

ABOUT THE AUTHOR

Joan Evans is a well-known nutritionist and has gained her certification as a weight loss expert at a very young age. During her early twenties, she is already very determined to make any effective material to reach out to everybody that body detoxification is essential as taking meal three times a day. Thus, she was able to come up with this great book.

Now, Joan Evans is an inspiration to those who want to lose weight, be healthy, and be more sexy and daring even during late forties.